Healthy Liver For Life And Cookbook: Breakfast and Snacks

Learn To Manage Your Nutrition With No Stress - Prevent Cirrhosis And Keep A Healthy Liver

Loren Allen

Healthy Liver For Life Cookbook

© Copyright 2021 by Loren Allen - All rights reserved.

The following Book is reproduced below with the goal of providing information that is as accurate and reliable as possible. Regardless, purchasing this Book can be seen as consent to the fact that both the publisher and the author of this book are in no way experts on the topics discussed within and that any recommendations or suggestions that are made herein are for entertainment purposes only. Professionals should be consulted as needed prior to undertaking any of the action endorsed herein.

This declaration is deemed fair and valid by both the American Bar Association and the Committee of Publishers Association and is legally binding throughout the United States.

Furthermore, the transmission, duplication, or reproduction of any of the following work including specific information will be considered an illegal act irrespective of if it is done electronically or in print. This extends to creating a secondary or tertiary copy of the work or a recorded copy and is only allowed with the express written consent from the Publisher. All additional right reserved.

Healthy Liver For Life Cookbook

The information in the following pages is broadly considered a truthful and accurate account of facts and as such, any inattention, use, or misuse of the information in question by the reader will render any resulting actions solely under their purview. There are no scenarios in which the publisher or the original author of this work can be in any fashion deemed liable for any hardship or damages that may befall them after undertaking information described herein.

Additionally, the information in the following pages is intended only for informational purposes and should thus be thought of as universal. As befitting its nature, it is presented without assurance regarding its prolonged validity or interim quality. Trademarks that are mentioned are done without written consent and can in no way be considered an endorsement from the trademark holder.

Table Of Contents

One Of The Most Vital Organs With More Than 500 Functions Known To Date	8
Tips For People With Liver Cirrhosis Disease	10
Functions Of The Liver - The Liver: Your Body's Most Important Muscle	17
Discovering the Stages of Liver Failure	23
Liver failure vs. liver disease	25
Stages of liver failure	26
Causes of liver failure	28
Symptoms of acute liver failure	31
Symptoms of chronic liver failure	31
Diagnosing liver failure	33
What are the treatment options for liver failure?	35
Preventing liver failure	37
Outlook	38

Orzo And Veggie Bowls	40
Eggplant Rollatini	42
Broccoli Omelette	44
Cherry Berry Bulgur Bowl	45
Gluten Free Pancakes	47
Slow-cooked Peppers Frittata	49
Veggie Omelet	51
Toxin Flush & Detox Salad	53
Chili Scramble	55
Couscous With Artichokes, Sun-dried Tomatoes And Feta	57
Tahini Pine Nuts Toast	59
Milk Scones	60
Vanilla Oats	62
Buckwheat Pancakes	64
Eggs And Veggies	66
Bacon Veggies Combo	68
Spicy Cucumbers	70
Raspberry Pudding	71

Onion Omelette	72
Spinach Wrap	73
Cauliflower Hash Brown Breakfast Bowl	76
Bacon, Vegetable And Parmesan Combo	78
Nectarine Pancakes	80
Herbed Spinach Frittata	81
Breakfast Tostadas	83
Pasta With Indian Lentils	86
Banana Pancakes	88
Almond Cream Cheese Bake	89
Baked Curried Apple Oatmeal Cups	91
Keto Egg Fast Snickerdoodle Crepes	93
Seeds And Lentils Oats	95
Mediterranean Egg Casserole	97
Red Pepper And Artichoke Frittata	102
Cinnamon Roll Oats	105
Cauliflower Couscous Salad	107
Mediterranean Egg-feta Scramble	109

Detox Porridge	111
Mexican Style Burritos	113
Stuffed Figs	115
Tapioca Pudding	117
Pumpkin Muffins	119
Snack	121
Za'atar Fries	121
Orange Salsa	123
Crazy Saganaki Shrimp	124
Apple Chips	126
Walnut & Spiced Apple Tonic	127
Raw Broccoli Poppers	128
Cod And Cabbage	130
Healthy Carrot & Shrimp	131
Spiced Toasted Almonds & Seed Mix	133
Conclusion	**135**

Healthy Liver For Life Cookbook

One Of The Most Vital Organs With More Than 500 Functions Known To Date

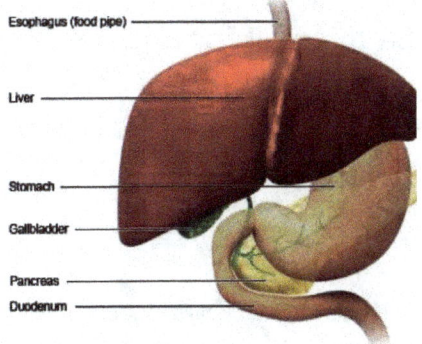

The liver is one of the most vital organs, with more than 500 functions known to date. If your organ's damage from cirrhosis means it can't efficiently perform its duty in getting nutrients out of food and into our bodies for use, a diet tailored specifically towards this ailment may help provide adequate nutrition without over-working what little function you have left. Research has shown that people who are suffering from hepatic diseases like hepatitis or cirrhosis are at risk for complications such as death if they don't receive enough nourishment (emphasis on protein) through their diets; so be sure not to skip meals!

Authors of a 2018 article in the Journal of Clinical Gastroenterology say that "dietary management of cirrhosis is not a one-size-fits-all approach but should be implemented earlier on in the treatment algorithm to improve the clinical prognosis of cirrhosis."

If you have liver cirrhosis, then it's important to stay on top of your diet. If not managed well enough, scarring will continue and worsen which can lead to a number of issues such as an increased risk for cancer or bleeding due to the organ being unable provide blood clotting capability.

If you're concerned about whether managing your diet is something that would be too much trouble for someone with hepatic impairment; don't worry - there are plenty of recipes out there available at any grocery store in most major cities! There should also be information readily available online if one need help finding their way through cooking healthy dishes easily without sacrificing taste.

Tips For People With Liver Cirrhosis Disease

Drinking alcohol and taking medications can cause liver disease to worsen. A healthy diet, like the Mediterranean Diet in combination with a few supplements will help you maintain your weight while limiting complications on the progression of liver disease. You want to avoid high-sugar beverages as well because they are very hard for your body's immune system when it is fighting an infection or just recovering from one!

In short, remember, eat food that is soft, avoid drinking alcohol, don't eat foods that are spicy.

1. Nutrition in Early Liver Cirrhosis Disease

Food

A healthy diet should consist of a variety of foods high in nutrients and vitamins. Healthy choices include fruit, vegetables, whole grains, lean protein sources such as chicken breast or tofu, unsalted nuts and seeds like walnuts or almonds for some crunchy texture to your meal on the side. Dairy products provide calcium needed for strong bones but be sure not to add too much fat with milk cheeses because they are higher in saturated fats than low-fat dairy options without cheese that will help keep you full longer after eating them - perfect before bedtime snacks! Keep sodium content lower by avoiding ketchup which is surprisingly one food containing large amounts of salt per serving size at 560mg/1 tbsp., pickles also contain an average 77% more

Selecting foods with healthy fats is important. Choosing unsaturated fats instead of saturated fats and trans fats is a good first step. Unsaturated fats:

- include monosaturated, polyunsaturated and Omega3 fatty acids

- come from plant sources and fish and include avocado, nuts, olive oil, canola oil and safflower oil

- foods high in Omega3 fatty acids include salmon, tuna and mackerel

Beverages

Drink water. Drinking too much sugar is bad for your body and may lead to weight gain or diabetes. Keep in mind that coffee can be good for you, but only up to three cups each day - any more than this could cause a variety of health problems including liver disease like cirrhosis! As always, it's important not to drink alcohol when the goal is improved liver health.

Vitamins and Minerals

Vitamins are the best way to keep you healthy, even if that's all you're eating is a variety of unhealthy foods. One exception would be in cases where someone has alcoholic liver disease and thiamine (vitamin B1), folic acid, and multivitamins should be taken- this includes vitamins B2 and B6 as well. If your diagnosis doesn't include hemochromatosis then vitamin C can also help prevent illness which may arise from an imbalance between iron absorption or retention levels due to genetics or autoimmune conditions such as celiac disease .

Vitamins provide much needed nutrients for many people who might not otherwise get them through their diet alone! An example would be those with alcohol related liver diseases; they

2. Nutrition in Advanced Liver Cirrhosis Disease

Food

Poor appetite, nausea and vomiting can lead to malnutrition in advanced liver disease (ALD). Loss of protein from decreased absorption or increased losses also contribute. Protein is not restricted even with ALD but you should avoid large amounts due the fact that your body does not store it well. Eating small meals more frequently may be better tolerated by an individual with ALD since they are much easier for their now-defunct liver to process than larger ones would be at one sitting time per day--this will also help keep them feeling full longer!

ALD causes the kidneys to hold sodium (salt) which then results in your body holding more fluid thus increasing ascites (swollen abdomen) and swelling of the hands, legs and feet. Your provider may ask that you restrict your sodium intake to 2000 mg or less (1 teaspoon of salt contains approximately 2300mg sodium). Sodium in all foods and beverages must be calculated into this amount. Reading sodium content on packaging will be necessary. You should remember that the sodium content on the package is for the serving size indicated on the label, not for the entire amount of the package. If you have chronic kidney disease, salt substitutes should be avoided because they are high in potassium.

Healthy Liver For Life Cookbook

Beverages

Your provider will tell you if or when to restrict your fluid intake with liver disease. The goal is 1500-2000 ml per day, but more than that can be prescribed by a doctor in order alleviate symptoms of feeling thirsty which could stem from taking diuretics (water pills). One way to keep track of how much water you drink for the whole day would be filling up one pitcher and every time we drink something take out an equivalent amount of water so it never goes below this limit! If on a restricted diet due to being on these medications, there are tricks such as drinking soup instead because they still count towards the daily total. Sugar-free frozen pops, sugar-free sour candy, sugar-free gelatin, sucking on lemon or lime slices and eating ice cold fruit and vegetables will help relieve thirst. Frozen grapes are a good option. Fluid from the sugar-free frozen pops and gelatin must be included in the daily allowance of fluid intake, as will the fluid in juicy fruit like watermelon.

Vitamins and Minerals

There is a fine line between not enough and too much when taking vitamin supplements. When you are sick, it may be difficult to know what the right amount of vitamins for your illness might be if you aren't sure of their effects on an already broken system. For example, excessive amounts can injure your liver which is at risk in this case because they have also been depleted from other illnesses such as Jaundice (yellow skin and eyes).

Fatigue, muscle weakness and twitches and cramps of your arms, hands and feet may indicate magnesium deficiency in ALD. Your provider may order a blood test to determine magnesium level and, if low, a supplement will be ordered. ALD may also cause a zinc deficiency. Signs of a zinc deficiency include decreased appetite, decreased ability to fight infection, diarrhea and hair loss. A zinc supplement may be ordered by your provider. Muscle cramps can also be relieved with drinking either regular or diet tonic water because of the quinine content. It is important not to drink more than 4 ounces per day because of the high sodium content.

Functions Of The Liver - The Liver: Your Body's Most Important Muscle

The liver is the largest organ in your body and without it life would be impossible. The liver's job includes filtering blood, maintaining healthy sugar levels, regulating clotting of blood (which prevents you from bleeding excessively), and performing hundreds more tasks that keep us alive. Located just under our ribs on the right side of our abdomen, this most important muscle helps fight infection by making new cells to replace dying ones!

Key Facts

The liver filters all of the blood in the body and breaks down poisonous substances, such as alcohol and drugs.

The liver also produces bile, a fluid that helps digest fats and carry away waste.

Healthy Liver For Life Cookbook

The liver consists of four lobes, which are each made up of eight sections and thousands of lobules (or small lobes).

Functions of the Liver

The liver is the body's trash compactor, producing essential blood sugars and nutrients. It also removes waste products from your bloodstream to provide you with a squeaky-clean circulatory system!

A lot of people might not be aware that their liver does so much work for them every day, but it really can't do everything without some help or support either - just like any other muscle in your body needs extra care when tired after working out. That said, there are healthy diet options to give yourself an energy boost so that this important organ doesn't have as tough a time performing its functions throughout the course of our 24 hour lifespan.

Albumin Production: Albumin is a protein that keeps fluids in the bloodstream from leaking into surrounding tissue. It also carries hormones, vitamins, and enzymes through the body.

Bile Production: Bile is a fluid that is critical to the digestion and absorption of fats in the small intestine.

Filters Blood: All the blood leaving the stomach and intestines passes through the liver, which removes toxins, byproducts, and other harmful substances.

Regulates Amino Acids: The production of proteins depend on amino acids. The liver makes sure amino acid levels in the bloodstream remain healthy.

Regulates Blood Clotting: Blood clotting coagulants are created using vitamin K, which can only be absorbed with the help of bile, a fluid the liver produces.

Resists Infections: As part of the filtering process, the liver also removes bacteria from the bloodstream.

Stores Vitamins and Minerals: The liver stores significant amounts of vitamins A, D, E, K, and B12, as well as iron and copper.

Processes Glucose: The liver removes excess glucose (sugar) from the bloodstream and stores it as glycogen. As needed, it can convert glycogen back into glucose.

Anatomy of the Liver

The liver is reddish-brown and shaped approximately like a cone or a wedge, with the small end above the spleen and stomach and the large end above the small intestine. The entire organ is located below the lungs in the right upper abdomen. It weighs between 3 and 3.5 pounds.

Structure

The liver is a large organ that consists of four lobes. The two larger, right lobe and left lobe are divided by the falciform ligament, which connects the liver to the abdominal wall. These segments can be further subdivided into eight smaller ones each with its own ducts for bile (a digestive fluid).

Parts

The following are some of the most important individual parts of the liver:

Common Hepatic Duct: A tube that carries bile out of the liver. It is formed from the intersection of the right and left hepatic ducts.

Falciform Ligament: A thin, fibrous ligament that separates the two lobes of the liver and connects it to the abdominal wall.

Glisson's Capsule: A layer of loose connective tissue that surrounds the liver and its related arteries and ducts.

Hepatic Artery: The main blood vessel that supplies the liver with oxygenated blood.

Hepatic Portal Vein: The blood vessel that carries blood from the gastrointestinal tract, gallbladder, pancreas, and spleen to the liver.

Lobes: The anatomical sections of the liver.

Lobules: Microscopic building blocks of the liver.

Peritoneum: A membrane covering the liver that forms the exterior.

Maintaining a Healthy Liver

Healthy Liver For Life Cookbook

The best way to avoid liver disease is by taking active steps towards a healthy life. The following are some recommendations that will help keep the liver functioning as it should:

Avoid Illicit Drugs: Illicit drugs are toxins that the liver must filter out. Taking these drugs can cause long-term damage.

Drink Alcohol Moderately: Alcohol must be broken down by the liver. While the liver can moderate amounts, excessive alcohol use can cause damage.

Exercise Regularly: A regular exercise routine will help promote general health for every organ, including the liver.

Eat Healthy Foods: Eating excessive fats can make it difficult for the liver to function and lead to fatty liver disease.

Practice Safe Sex: Use protection to avoid sexually transmitted diseases such as hepatitis C.

Vaccinate: Especially when traveling, get appropriate vaccinations against hepatitis A and B, as well as diseases such as malaria and yellow fever, which grow in the liver.

Discovering the Stages of Liver Failure

Liver failure is a life-threatening emergency. The two main types of liver failures are acute or chronic and it can either come on quickly, like when one has an infection that leads to increased alcohol abuse or if you're born with certain genetics (such as hemochromatosis), whereas the other type occurs gradually over time in some people who may not have any risks factors for developing their disease but just develop them due to lifestyle choices.

Acute liver failure suddenly comes on while chronic cases happen slowly over weeks/months so they're easier treated before serious damage happens; however, this doesn't mean your symptoms will go away because there's no cure--only treatments--and many sufferers don't know about early signs which could be monitored.

The liver is an important part of the body. It can be damaged and not work properly. The damage can happen in stages that get worse over time.

Stages of liver failure

Inflammation. In this early stage, the liver is enlarged or inflamed.

Fibrosis. Scar tissue begins to replace healthy tissue in the inflamed liver.

Cirrhosis. Severe scarring has built up, making it difficult for the liver to function properly.

End-stage liver disease (ESLD). Liver function has deteriorated to the point where the damage can't be reversed other than with a liver transplant.

Liver cancer. The development and multiplication of unhealthy cells in the liver can occur at any stage of liver failure, although people with cirrhosis are more at risk.

Liver failure vs. liver disease

The liver is one of the most important organs in your body. There are many different types of diseases that can affect it, but two specific ones to watch out for are degenerative and acute hepatitis. The first usually causes damage over time while the latter often occurs quickly due to rapid infection or injury from an outside source like alcohol abuse or a car accident. These conditions result in inflammation, pain, swelling and even death if left untreated! It's good you know what these look like so when they come up on your medical tests you'll be able to react appropriately instead of waiting around until something more serious happens again later down the line.

Stages of liver failure

Damage from liver disease can happen in stages. The damage goes up and it makes the liver not work as well.

Inflammation

In this early stage, your liver becomes swollen or inflamed. Many people with this condition do not have symptoms. If it continues for a long time, your liver can be permanently damaged.

Fibrosis

Fibrosis is inflammation of the liver. This can happen when the liver starts to scar.

The scar tissue that's generated in this stage replaces healthy liver tissue. But the scarred tissue can't do what the healthy tissue did. It can start to affect your liver's ability to work right.

Fibrosis is hard to notice because there are not usually any symptoms.

Cirrhosis

When you have cirrhosis, your liver is damaged. That means it doesn't work as well.

When you first get liver disease, you may not have any symptoms. But now, you might start to feel bad.

End-stage liver disease (ESLD)

People with ESLD have a disease called cirrhosis. This means that the liver has been damaged.

ESLD is associated with complications such as ascites and hepatic encephalopathy. It can't be reversed unless you get a liver transplant.

Liver cancer

Cancer is when cells in your body are not healthy. If you have cancer in your liver, it is called primary liver cancer.

Although it can happen at any stage of liver failure, people with cirrhosis are more likely to get liver cancer.

Some common symptoms of liver cancer include:

- unexplained weight loss
- abdominal pain or swelling
- loss of appetite or feeling full after eating a small amount of food
- nausea or vomiting
- yellowing of the skin and eyes (jaundice)
- skin itching

Causes of liver failure

The cause of liver failure can depend on the type of liver failure — acute or chronic.

Causes of acute liver failure

Acute liver failure occurs quickly. It can be caused by many things, but sometimes the exact cause is unknown.. Some possible causes include:

- A viral infection happens when a virus enters the body. There are three viruses that can cause infections: hepatitis A, B, or E.
- A person might overdose on acetaminophen (Tylenol) if they take too much.
- There are many different reactions to prescription medicines. For example, some people might have a reaction when they use antibiotics, NSAIDs or anti-epileptic drugs.
- Reactions to herbal supplements, such as ma huang and kava kava.
- metabolic conditions, such as Wilson's disease
- autoimmune conditions are when your body attacks itself. For example, there is autoimmune hepatitis.
- If you have the condition where the veins of your liver are affected, like Budd-Chiari syndrome, then it is important to eat less fat.
- Exposure to toxins can happen in the workplace or when you eat a bad mushroom.

Causes of chronic liver failure

Liver failure happens when a person's liver gets hurt over time. This can lead to cirrhosis, which is when there is too much scar tissue on the liver and it stops working right.

Some examples of possible causes of cirrhosis include:

- chronic hepatitis B or C infection
- Alcohol-related liver disease (ARLD) is a disease that can happen when you drink alcohol. It happens in your liver.
- Nonalcoholic fatty liver disease means that someone has a lot of fat in their liver and they do not drink alcohol.
- autoimmune hepatitis
- Diseases that affect your bile duct can be very bad. They are called cholangitis.

Symptoms of acute liver failure

Acute liver failure can happen to people who do not have a condition in their liver. This is an emergency and people should see a doctor when they have symptoms that are like acute liver failure.

The symptoms of acute liver failure can include:

- feeling unwell (malaise)
- feeling tired or sleepy
- nausea or vomiting
- abdominal pain or swelling
- yellowing of the skin and eyes (jaundice)
- feeling confused or disoriented

Symptoms of chronic liver failure

Some symptoms of chronic liver failure are early symptoms and some are more advanced. Early symptoms may include:

- feeling tired or fatigued
- loss of appetite
- nausea or vomiting
- mild abdominal discomfort or pain

Some symptoms that might mean you have a liver problem are:

- yellowing of the skin and eyes (jaundice)
- easy bruising or bleeding
- feeling confused or disoriented
- buildup of fluid in your abdomen, arms, or legs
- darkening of your urine
- severe skin itching

Diagnosing liver failure

To diagnose liver failure, your doctor will start by taking your medical history and performing a physical examination. They may then perform additional tests to rule out other causes of symptoms such as: blood work-up for anemia or anaemia; chest X-ray to look at the lungs and heart health; EKG for an irregular heartbeat (arrhythmia); urinalysis looking at kidney function along with electrolytes in urine samples.; imaging scans like ultrasounds or CTs which can visualize different parts of our body.

You might also have some generalized pain around the abdomen area that you'll need to mention on this list too!

- A **liver blood test** is a test to see how your liver is working. There are different proteins and enzymes in the blood, and these can tell.
- **Other blood tests.** Your doctor can do a blood test to see if you have any problems in your liver. There are many different tests that they can do.
- **Imaging tests.** Ultrasound, CT scan, and MRI can help your doctor to see your liver.
- **Biopsy.** Taking a tissue sample of your liver can help your doctor see if there is scar tissue or other reasons for your condition.

What are the treatment options for liver failure?

The liver is important for our body. We need it to help us do things like digest food, and if it doesn't work, then we will have a problem. If there is something going wrong with our liver, then we might have to take medicine or get surgery so that the damage can stop happening.

For example, antiviral medications can be used to treat a viral hepatitis infection, or immune suppressing medication can be given to treat autoimmune hepatitis.

Lifestyle changes may also be recommended as a part of your treatment. These can include things like abstaining from alcohol, losing weight, or avoiding the use of certain medications.

The American Liver Foundation estimates that a large percentage of the damage to your liver can be reversed, if caught and treated. If not, this may lead to cirrhosis or ESLD which is often irreversible but sometimes slows down progression.

What about acute liver failure?

Acute liver failure is often treated in the intensive care unit of a hospital. Supportive care can be given to help stabilize your condition and control any complications during treatment and recovery from acute liver failure.

A medication overdose or reaction may also lead you to receive drugs that reverse its effects, while a potential indication for transplantation may exist for some people with this type of serious medical emergency due to their severe illness severity, which could even progress into coma if left untreated too long!

Preventing liver failure

You can help to prevent liver failure by making lifestyle changes. If you make them, your liver will be happy and healthy. Here are some tips for improving liver health:

- Drink alcohol in moderation, and never mix medications with alcohol.
- Take medications only when needed, and carefully follow any dosing instructions.
- Don't mix medications without first consulting your doctor.
- To maintain a healthy weight, there is a connection to liver disease.
- Get vaccinated against hepatitis A and B.
- Be sure to have regular physicals with your doctor during which they perform liver blood tests.

Outlook

Liver failure is when your liver can't function properly. It can be either acute or chronic, and in the later stages of life it may require a transplant to save lives. Liver deterioration could have been caused by alcoholism, hepatitis-C infection, cancer treatment side effects such as chemotherapy drugs that damage the healthy cells along with tumor cells; or even radiation for kidney stones where some parts of belly will get more exposed than others due to increased urination which was previously being handled by kidneys before they were damaged from stone disease - you name it! In any case though whether its just one factor like alcohol abuse leading up to cirrhosis and then eventually hepatocellular carcinoma (liver cancer) if untreated through surgery followed.

People who are diagnosed with liver disease are often monitored throughout their life to make sure that their condition isn't worsening or causing further liver damage. If you have concerns about liver health or about liver failure, be sure to talk to your doctor.

Orzo And Veggie Bowls

Servings: 4

Cooking Time: 10 Minutes

Ingredients:

- 2 and ½ cups whole-wheat orzo, cooked
- 14 ounces canned cannellini beans, drained and rinsed
- 1 yellow bell pepper, cubed
- 1 green bell pepper, cubed
- A pinch of salt and black pepper
- 3 tomatoes, cubed
- 1 red onion, chopped
- 1 cup mint, chopped
- 2 cups feta cheese, crumbled
- 2 tablespoons olive oil
- ¼ cup lemon juice
- 1 tablespoon lemon zest, grated
- 1 cucumber, cubed
- 1 and ¼ cup kalamata olives, pitted and sliced
- 3 garlic cloves, minced

Directions:

In a salad bowl, combine the orzo with the beans, bell peppers and the rest of the ingredients, toss, divide the mix between plates and serve for breakfas

Nutrition:

calories 411, fat 17, fiber 13, carbs 51, protein 14

Eggplant Rollatini

Servings:4

Cooking Time:25 Minutes

Ingredients:

- 1 eggplant
- 12 oz. ricotta cheese
- 2 oz. mozzarella cheese
- 1 can tomatoes
- ¼ tsp salt
- 2 tablespoons seasoning

Directions:

- Lay the eggplant on a baking sheet
- Roast at 350 F for 12-15 minutes
- In a bowl combine mozzarella, seasoning, tomatoes, ricotta cheese and salt
- Add cheese mixture to the eggplant and roll
- Place the rolls into a baking dish and bake for another 10-12 minutes
- When ready remove from the oven and serve

Nutrition:

35g carbs 30g fat 20g protein 460 Calories

Broccoli Omelette

Servings:1

Cooking Time:10 Minutes

Ingredients:

- 2 eggs
- ¼ tsp salt
- ¼ tsp black pepper
- 1 tablespoon olive oil
- ¼ cup cheese
- ¼ tsp basil
- 1 cup broccoli

Directions:

- In a bowl combine all ingredients together and mix well
- In a skillet heat olive oil and pour the egg mixture
- Cook for 1-2 minutes per side
- When ready remove omelette from the skillet and serve

Nutrition:

50g carbs 11g fat 10g protein 320 Calories

Cherry Berry Bulgur Bowl

Servings:4

Cooking Time:15 Minutes

Ingredients:

- 1 cup medium-grind bulgur
- 2 cups water
- Pinch salt
- 1 cup halved and pitted cherries or 1 cup canned cherries, drained
- ½ cup raspberries
- ½ cup blackberries
- 1 tablespoon cherry jam
- 2 cups plain whole-milk yogurt

Directions:

1. Mix the bulgur, water, and salt in a medium saucepan. Do this in a medium heat. Bring to a boil.
2. Reduce the heat to low and simmer, partially covered, for 12 to 15 minutes or until the bulgur is almost tender. Cover, and let stand for 5 minutes to finish cooking do this after removing the pan from the heat.
3. While the bulgur is cooking, combine the raspberries and blackberries in a medium bowl. Stir the cherry jam into the fruit.
4. When the bulgur is tender, divide among four bowls. Top each bowl with ½ cup of yogurt and an equal amount of the berry mixture and serve.

Nutrition:

Calories: 242; Total fat: 6g; Saturated fat: 3g; Sodium: 85mg; Phosphorus: 237mg; Potassium: 438mg; Carbohydrates: 44g; Fiber: 7g; Protein: 9g; Sugar: 13g

Gluten Free Pancakes

Servings: 3

Cooking Time:

Ingredients:

- 1 cup almond flour
- 1/4 cup coconut flour
- 1/3 cup unsweetened almond milk
- 3 large eggs
- 1/4 cup olive oil
- 1 teaspoon baking powder
- 1 1/2 teaspoons vanilla extract
- 1 tablespoon raw honey
- 1 cup fresh blueberries for serving

Directions:

1. In a large bowl, whisk together all the ingredients until very smooth. Heat a pan and then add in oil; drop about three tablespoons of batter into the pan and cook for about 2 minutes. flip over and cook for 2 minutes more or until lightly browned on both sides. Repeat with the remaining batter.
2. Serve topped with fresh blueberries

Nutrition:

242 Calories 7g Carbs 19g Fat 12g Protein

Slow-cooked Peppers Frittata

Servings: 4

Cooking Time: 60 Minutes

Ingredients:

- ½ cup almond milk
- 8 eggs, whisked
- Salt and black pepper to the taste
- 1 teaspoon oregano, dried
- 1 and ½ cups roasted peppers, chopped
- ½ cup red onion, chopped
- 4 cups baby arugula
- 1 cup goat cheese, crumbled
- Cooking spray

Directions:

- In a bowl, combine the eggs with salt, pepper and the oregano and whisk.
- Grease your slow cooker with the cooking spray, arrange the peppers and the remaining ingredients inside and pour the eggs mixture over them.
- Put the lid on and cook on Low for 3 hours.
- Divide the frittata between plates and serve.

Nutrition:

calories 259, fat 20.2, fiber 1, carbs 4.4, protein 16.3

Veggie Omelet

Servings:3

Cooking Time:20 Minutes

Ingredients:

- 3 egg whites
- 1 egg
- 1/2 teaspoon extra-virgin olive oil
- 1/8 teaspoon red pepper flakes
- 1/8 teaspoon ground nutmeg
- 1/8 teaspoon garlic powder
- A Pinch of salt
- 1/8 teaspoon ground black pepper
- 1/2 cup sliced fresh mushrooms
- 2 tablespoons chopped red bell pepper
- 1/4 cup chopped green onion
- 1/2 cup chopped tomato
- 1 cup chopped fresh spinach

Directions:

- In a large bowl, whisk together egg whites, egg, garlic powder, red pepper flakes, nutmeg, salt and pepper until well blended.
- Heat olive oil in a skillet over medium heat; add green onion, mushrooms and belle pepper and cook for about 5 minutes or until tender; stir in tomato and egg mixture and cook for about 5 minutes per side or until egg is set. Slice and serve hot.

Nutrition:

283.6 Calories 11.5g fat 31g carbs 10.9g protein

Toxin Flush & Detox Salad

Servings:3

Cooking Time:10 Minutes

Ingredients:

- For the salad:
- 2 cups broccoli florets
- 2 cups red cabbage, thinly sliced
- 2 cups chopped kale
- 1 cup grated carrot
- 1 red bell pepper, sliced into strips
- 2 avocados, diced
- 1/2 cup chopped parsley
- 1 cup walnuts
- 1 tablespoon sesame seeds
- For the dressing:
- 2 teaspoons gluten-free mustard
- 1 tablespoon freshly grated ginger
- 1/2 cup fresh lemon juice
- 1/3 cup grapeseed oil
- 1 teaspoon raw honey
- 1/4 teaspoon salt

Directions:

- In a blender, blend all the dressing ingredients until well blended; set aside.
- In a salad bowl, mix broccoli, cabbage, kale, carrots and bell pepper; pour the dressing over the salad and toss until well coated.
- Add diced avocado, parsley, walnuts and sesame seed; toss again to coat and serve.

Nutrition:

283.6 Calories 11.5g fat 31g carbs 10.9g protein

Chili Scramble

Servings: 4

Cooking Time: 13 Minutes

Ingredients:

- 3 tomatoes
- 4 eggs
- ¼ teaspoon of sea salt
- ½ chili pepper, chopped
- 1 tablespoon butter
- 1 cup water, for cooking

Directions:

- Pour water in the saucepan and bring it to boil.
- Then remove water from the heat and add tomatoes.
- Let the tomatoes stay in the hot water for 2-3 minutes.
- After this, remove the tomatoes from water and peel them.
- Place butter in the pan and melt it.
- Add chopped chili pepper and fry it for 3 minutes over the medium heat.
- Then chop the peeled tomatoes and add into the chili peppers.
- Cook the vegetables for 5 minutes over the medium heat. Stir them from time to time.
- After this, add sea salt and crack then eggs.
- Stir (scramble) the eggs well with the help of the fork and cook them for 3 minutes over the medium heat.

Nutrition:

calories 105, fat 7.4, fiber 1.1, carbs 4, protein 6.4

Couscous With Artichokes, Sun-dried Tomatoes And Feta

Servings: 4

Cooking Time:

Ingredients:

- 3 cups chicken breast, cooked, chopped
- 2 1/3 cups water, divided
- 2 jars (6-ounces each) marinated artichoke hearts, undrained
- 1/4 teaspoon black pepper, freshly ground
- 1/2 cup tomatoes, sun-dried
- 1/2 cup (2 ounces) feta cheese, crumbled
- 1 cup flat-leaf parsley, fresh, chopped
- 1 3/4 cups whole-wheat Israeli couscous, uncooked
- 1 can (14 1/2 ounces) vegetable broth

Directions:

- In a microwavable bowl, combine 2 cups of the water and the tomatoes. Microwave on HIGH for about 3 minutes or until the water boils. When water is boiling, remove from the microwave, cover, and let stand for about 3 minutes or until the tomatoes are soft; drain, chop, and set aside.
- In a large saucepan, place the vegetable broth and the remaining 1/3 cup of water; bring to boil. Stir in the couscous, cover, reduce heat, and simmer for about 8 minutes or until tender. Remove the pan from the heat; add the tomatoes and the remaining ingredients. Stir to combine.

Nutrition:

419 Cal, 14.1 g total fat (3.9 g sat. fat, 0.8 g poly. Fat, 1.4 g mono), 64 mg chol., 677 mg sodium, 42.5 g carb., 2.6 g fiber, 30.2 g protein.

Tahini Pine Nuts Toast

Servings:4

Cooking Time:10 Minutes

Ingredients:

- 2 whole wheat bread slices, toasted
- 1 teaspoon water
- 1 tablespoon tahini paste
- 2 teaspoons feta cheese, crumbled
- Juice of ½ lemon
- 2 teaspoons pine nuts
- A pinch of black pepper

Directions:

- In a bowl, mix the tahini with the water and the lemon juice, whisk really well and spread over the toasted bread slices.
- Top each serving with the remaining ingredients and serve for breakfast.

Nutrition:

calories 142, fat 7.6, fiber 2.7, carbs 13.7, protein 5.8

Milk Scones

Servings: 4

Cooking Time: 10 Minutes

Ingredients:

- ½ cup wheat flour, whole grain
- 1 teaspoon baking powder
- 1 tablespoon butter, melted
- 1 teaspoon vanilla extract
- 1 egg, beaten
- ¾ teaspoon salt
- 3 tablespoons milk
- 1 teaspoon vanilla sugar

Directions:

1. In the mixing bowl combine together wheat flour, baking powder, butter, vanilla extract, and egg. Add salt and knead the soft and non-sticky dough. Add more flour if needed.
2. Then make the log from the dough and cut it into the triangles.
3. Line the tray with baking paper.
4. Arrange the dough triangles on the baking paper and transfer in the preheat to the 360F oven.
5. Cook the scones for 10 minutes or until they are light brown.
6. After this, chill the scones and brush with milk and sprinkle with vanilla sugar.

Nutrition:

calories 112, fat 4.4, fiber 0.5, carbs 14.3, protein 3.4

Vanilla Oats

Servings:4

Cooking Time:10 Minutes

Ingredients:

- ½ cup rolled oats
- 1 cup milk
- 1 teaspoon vanilla extract
- 1 teaspoon ground cinnamon
- 2 teaspoon honey
- 2 tablespoons Plain yogurt
- 1 teaspoon butter

Directions:

- Pour milk in the saucepan and bring it to boil.
- Add rolled oats and stir well.
- Close the lid and simmer the oats for 5 minutes over the medium heat. The cooked oats will absorb all milk.
- Then add butter and stir the oats well.
- In the separated bowl, whisk together Plain yogurt with honey, cinnamon, and vanilla extract.
- Transfer the cooked oats in the serving bowls.
- Top the oats with the yogurt mixture in the shape of the whe

Nutrition:

calories 243, fat 20.2, fiber 1, carbs 2.8, protein 13.3

Buckwheat Pancakes

Servings: 3

Cooking Time: 15 Minutes

Ingredients:

- 1/2 cup buckwheat flour
- 2 ripe bananas
- 2 tablespoons olive
- 2 tablespoons water
- 1 teaspoon ground cinnamon
- 1 teaspoon vanilla extract
- 1/2 teaspoon baking soda
- 2 teaspoons apple cider vinegar
- 1/4 cup fresh blueberries for serving

Directions:

- Preheat your oven to 350 degrees.
- Add the ripe banana to a large bowl and mash until smooth; whisk in ground buckwheat flour, water, oil, vanilla, vinegar, cinnamon and baking powder until well combined.
- Heat a skillet over medium heat; add in oil and heat until hot but not smoky; add in about a quarter cup of batter and spread to cover the bottom of the pan.
- Cook for about 2 minutes and then flip to cook the other side for about 1 minute or until browned.
- Serve right away topped with fresh blueberries.

Nutrition:

242 Calories 25g carbs 12g fat 13g protein

Eggs And Veggies

Servings: 4

Cooking Time: 10 Minutes

Ingredients:

- 2 tomatoes, chopped
- 2 eggs, beaten
- 1 bell pepper, chopped
- 1 teaspoon tomato paste
- ¼ cup of water
- 1 teaspoon butter
- ½ white onion, diced
- ½ teaspoon chili flakes
- 1/3 teaspoon sea salt

Directions:

- Put butter in the pan and melt it.
- Add bell pepper and cook it for 3 minutes over the medium heat. Stir it from time to time.
- After this, add diced onion and cook it for 2 minutes more.
- Stir the vegetables and add tomatoes.
- Cook them for 5 minutes over the medium-low heat.
- Then add water and tomato paste. Stir well.
- Add beaten eggs, chili flakes, and sea salt.
- Stir well and cook menemen for 4 minutes over the medium-low heat.
- The cooked meal should be half runny.

Nutrition:

calories 67, fat 3.4, fiber 1.5, carbs 6.4, protein 3.8

Bacon Veggies Combo

Servings: 4

Cooking Time: 35 Minutes

Ingredients:

- ½ green bell pepper, seeded and chopped
- 2 bacon slices
- ¼ cup Parmesan Cheese
- ½ tablespoon mayonnaise
- 1 scallion, chopped

Directions:

1. Preheat the oven to 375 degrees F and grease a baking dish.
2. Place bacon slices on the baking dish and top with mayonnaise, bell peppers, scallions and Parmesan Cheese.
3. Transfer in the oven and bake for about 25 minutes.
4. Dish out to serve immediately or refrigerate for about 2 days wrapped in a plastic sheet for meal preparation ping.

Nutrition:

Calories: 197 Fat: 13.8g Carbohydrates: 4.7g
Protein: 14.3g Sugar: 1.9g Sodium: 662mg

Spicy Cucumbers

Servings:7

Cooking Time:20 Minutes

Ingredients:

- 2 cucumbers
- 1 cup Greek yogurt
- 1 garlic clove
- 1 tsp paprika
- 1 tsp dill
- 1 tsp chili powder

Directions:

1. In a bowl combine all ingredients together except cucumbers
2. Cut the cucumbers into rounds and scoot out the inside
3. Fill each cucumber with the spicy mixture
4. When ready sprinkle paprika and serve

Nutrition:

3g carbs 10g fat 12g protein 165 Calories

Raspberry Pudding

Servings:2

Cooking Time:30 Minutes

Ingredients:

- ½ cup raspberries
- 2 teaspoons maple syrup
- 1 ½ cup Plain yogurt
- ¼ teaspoon ground cardamom
- 1/3 cup Chia seeds, dried

Directions:

1. Mix up together Plain yogurt with maple syrup and ground cardamom.
2. Add Chia seeds. Stir it gently.
3. Put the yogurt in the serving glasses and top with the raspberries.
4. Refrigerate the breakfast for at least 30 minutes or overnight.

Nutrition:

calories 303, fat 11.2, fiber 11.8, carbs 33.2, protein 15.5

Onion Omelette

Servings:1

Cooking Time:10 Minutes

Ingredients:

- 2 eggs
- ¼ tsp salt
- ¼ tsp black pepper
- 1 tablespoon olive oil
- ¼ cup cheese
- ¼ tsp basil
- 1 cup red onion

Directions:

1. In a bowl combine all ingredients together and mix well
2. In a skillet heat olive oil and pour the egg mixture
3. Cook for 1-2 minutes per side
4. When ready remove omelette from the skillet and serve

Nutrition:

50g carbs 11g fat 10g protein 320 Calories

Spinach Wrap

Servings: 4

Cooking Time: 10 Minutes

Ingredients:

- 4 pieces (10-inch) spinach wraps (or whole wheat tortilla or sun-dried tomato wraps)
- 1 pound chicken tenders
- 1 cup cucumber, chopped
- 3 tablespoons extra-virgin olive oil
- 1 medium tomato, chopped
- 1/3 cup couscous, whole-wheat
- 2 teaspoons garlic, minced
- 1/4 teaspoon salt, divided
- 1/4 teaspoon freshly ground pepper
- 1/4 cup lemon juice
- 1/2 cup water
- 1/2 cup fresh mint, chopped
- 1 cup fresh parsley, chopped

Directions:

1. In a small saucepan, pour the water and bring to a boil. Stir in the couscous, remove pan from heat, cover, and allow to stand for 5 minutes, then fluff using a fork; set aside.
2. Meanwhile, in a small mixing bowl, combine the mint, parsley, oil, lemon juice, garlic, 1/8 teaspoon of the salt, and the pepper.
3. In a medium mixing bowl, toss the chicken with the 1 tablespoon of the mint mixture and the remaining 1/8 teaspoon of salt.
4. Place the chicken mixture into a large non-stick skillet; cook for about 3-5 minutes each side, or until heated through. Remove from the skillet, allow to cool enough to handle, and cut into bite-sized pieces.
5. Stir the remaining mint mixture, the cucumber, and the tomato into the couscous.
6. Spread about 3/4 cup of the couscous mix onto each wrap and divide the chicken between the wraps, roll like a burrito, tucking the sides in to hold to secure the ingredients in. Cut in halves and serv

Nutrition:

479 Cal, 17 g total fat (3 g sat. fat, 11 g mono), 67 mg chol., 653 mg sodium, 382 pot., 49 g carb.,5 g fiber, 15 g protein

Cauliflower Hash Brown Breakfast Bowl

Servings:2

Cooking Time:30 Minutes

Ingredients:

- 1 tablespoon lemon juice
- 1 egg
- 1 avocado
- 1 teaspoon garlic powder
- 2 tablespoons extra virgin olive oil
- 2 oz mushrooms, sliced
- ½ green onion, chopped
- ¼ cup salsa
- ¾ cup cauliflower rice
- ½ small handful baby spinach
- Salt and black pepper, to taste

Directions:

Healthy Liver For Life Cookbook

1. Mash together avocado, lemon juice, garlic powder, salt and black pepper in a small bowl.
2. Whisk eggs, salt and black pepper in a bowl and keep aside.
3. Heat half of olive oil over medium heat in a skillet and add mushrooms.
4. Sauté for about 3 minutes and season with garlic powder, salt, and pepper.
5. Sauté for about 2 minutes and dish out in a bowl.
6. Add rest of the olive oil and add cauliflower, garlic powder, salt and pepper.
7. Sauté for about 5 minutes and dish out.
8. Return the mushrooms to the skillet and add green onions and baby spinach.
9. Sauté for about 30 seconds and add whisked eggs.
10. Sauté for about 1 minute and scoop on the sautéed cauliflower hash browns.
11. Top with salsa and mashed avocado and serve

Nutrition:

Calories: 400 Carbs: 15.8g Fats: 36.7g Proteins: 8g Sodium: 288mg Sugar: 4.2g

Bacon, Vegetable And Parmesan Combo

Servings:2

Cooking Time:30 Minutes

Ingredients:

- 2 slices of bacon, thick-cut
- ½ tbsp mayonnaise
- ½ of medium green bell pepper, deseeded, chopped
- 1 scallion, chopped
- ¼ cup grated Parmesan cheese
- 1 tbsp olive oil

- Switch on the oven, then set its temperature to 375°F and let it preheat.
- Meanwhile, take a baking dish, grease it with oil, and add slices of bacon in it.
- Spread mayonnaise on top of the bacon, then top with bell peppers and scallions, sprinkle with Parmesan cheese and bake for about 25 minutes until cooked thoroughly.
- When done, take out the baking dish and serve immediately.
- For meal preparation ping, wrap bacon in a plastic sheet and refrigerate for up to 2 days.
- When ready to eat, reheat bacon in the microwave and then serve

Nutrition:

Calories 197, Total Fat 13.8g, Total Carbs 4.7g, Protein 14.3g, Sugar 1.9g, Sodium 662mg

Nectarine Pancakes

Servings: 4

Cooking Time: 30 Minutes

Ingredients:

- 1 cup whole wheat flour
- ¼ tsp baking soda
- ¼ tsp baking powder
- 1 cup nectarines
- 2 eggs
- 1 cup milk

Directions:

1. In a bowl combine all ingredients together and mix well
2. In a skillet heat olive oil
3. Pour ¼ of the batter and cook each pancake for 1-2 minutes per side
4. When ready remove from heat and serve

Nutrition:

7g carbs 14g fat 15g protein 210 Calories

Herbed Spinach Frittata

Servings:4

Cooking Time:20 Minutes

Ingredients:

- 5 eggs, beaten
- 1 cup fresh spinach
- 2 oz Parmesan, grated
- 1/3 cup cherry tomatoes
- ½ teaspoon dried oregano
- 1 teaspoon dried thyme
- 1 teaspoon olive oi

Directions:

1. Chop the spinach into the tiny pieces and or use a blender.
2. Then combine together chopped spinach with eggs, dried oregano and thyme.
3. Add Parmesan and stir frittata mixture with the help of the fork.
4. Brush the springform pan with olive oil and pour the egg mixture inside.
5. Cut the cherry tomatoes into the halves and place them over the egg mixture.
6. Preheat the oven to 360F.
7. Bake the frittata for 20 minutes or until it is solid.
8. Chill the cooked breakfast till the room temperature and slice into the servings

Nutrition:

calories 140, fat 9.8, fiber 0.5, carbs 2.1, protein 11.9

Breakfast Tostadas

Servings:6

Cooking Time:30 Minutes

Ingredients:

- ½ white onion, diced
- 1 tomato, chopped
- 1 cucumber, chopped
- 1 tablespoon fresh cilantro, chopped
- ½ jalapeno pepper, chopped
- 1 tablespoon lime juice
- 6 corn tortillas
- 1 tablespoon canola oil
- 2 oz Cheddar cheese, shredded
- ½ cup white beans, canned, drained
- 6 eggs
- ½ teaspoon butter
- ½ teaspoon Sea salt

Directions:

1. Make Pico de Galo: in the salad bowl combine together diced white onion, tomato, cucumber, fresh cilantro, and jalapeno pepper.
2. Then add lime juice and a ½ tablespoon of canola oil. Mix up the mixture well. Pico de Galo is cooked.
3. After this, preheat the oven to 390F.
4. Line the tray with baking paper.
5. Arrange the corn tortillas on the baking paper and brush with remaining canola oil from both sides.
6. Bake the tortillas for 10 minutes or until they start to be crunchy.
7. Chill the cooked crunchy tortillas well.
8. Meanwhile, toss the butter in the skillet.
9. Crack the eggs in the melted butter and sprinkle them with sea salt.
10. Fry the eggs until the egg whites become white (cooked). Approximately for 3-5 minutes over the medium heat.
11. After this, mash the beans until you get puree texture.
12. Spread the bean puree on the corn tortillas.
13. Add fried eggs.
14. Then top the eggs with Pico de Galo and shredded Cheddar cheese

Nutrition:

Calories 246, fat 11.1, fiber 4.7, carbs 24.5, protein 13.7

Pasta With Indian Lentils

Servings:6

Cooking Time:5 Minutes

Ingredients:

- ¼-½ cup fresh cilantro (chopped)
- 3 cups water
- 2 small dry red peppers (whole)
- 1 teaspoon turmeric
- 1 teaspoon ground cumin
- 2-3 cloves garlic (minced)
- 1 can diced tomatoes (w/juice)
- 1 large onion (chopped)
- ½ cup dry lentils (rinsed)
- ½ cup orzo or tiny pasta

Directions:

1. Combine all ingredients in the skillet except for the cilantro then boil on medium-high heat.
2. Ensure to cover and slightly reduce heat to medium-low and simmer until pasta is tender for about 35 minutes.
3. Afterwards, take out the chili peppers then add cilantro and top it with low-fat sour cream.

Nutrition:

Calories: 175; Carbs: 40g; Protein: 3g; Fats: 2g; Phosphorus: 139mg; Potassium: 513mg; Sodium: 61mg

Banana Pancakes

Servings:4

Cooking Time:20 Minutes

Ingredients:

- 1 cup whole wheat flour
- ¼ tsp baking soda
- ¼ tsp baking powder
- 1 cup mashed banana
- 2 eggs
- 1 cup milk

Directions:

1. In a bowl combine all ingredients together and mix well
2. In a skillet heat olive oil
3. Pour ¼ of the batter and cook each pancake for 1-2 minutes per side
4. When ready remove from heat and serve

Nutrition:

7g carbs 14g fat 15g protein 210 Calories

Almond Cream Cheese Bake

Servings: 4

Cooking Time: 60 Minutes

Ingredients:

- 1 cup cream cheese
- 4 tablespoons honey
- 1 oz almonds, chopped
- ½ teaspoon vanilla extract
- 3 eggs, beaten
- 1 tablespoon semolina

Directions:

1. Put beaten eggs in the mixing bowl.
2. Add cream cheese, semolina, and vanilla extract.
3. Blend the mixture with the help of the hand mixer until it is fluffy.
4. After this, add chopped almonds and mix up the mass well.
5. Transfer the cream cheese mash in the non-sticky baking mold.
6. Flatten the surface of the cream cheese mash well.
7. Preheat the oven to 325F.
8. Cook the breakfast for 2 hours.
9. The meal is cooked when the surface of the mash is light brown.
10. Chill the cream cheese mash little and sprinkle with honey

Nutrition:

calories 352, fat 27.1, fiber 1, carbs 22.6, protein 10.4

Baked Curried Apple Oatmeal Cups

Servings:6

Cooking Time:20 Minutes

Ingredients:

- 3½ cups old-fashioned oats
- 3 tablespoons brown sugar
- 2 teaspoons of your preferred curry powder
- ⅛ teaspoon salt
- 1 cup unsweetened almond milk
- 1 cup unsweetened applesauce
- 1 teaspoon vanilla
- ½ cup chopped walnuts

Directions:

1. Preheat the oven to 375°F. Then spray a 12-cup muffin tin with baking spray then set aside.
2. Combine the oats, brown sugar, curry powder, and salt, and mix in a medium bowl.
3. Mix together the milk, applesauce, and vanilla in a small bowl,
4. Stir the liquid ingredients into the dry ingredients and mix until just combined. Stir in the walnuts.
5. Using a scant ⅓ cup for each divide the mixture among the muffin cups.
6. Bake this for 18 to 20 minutes until the oatmeal is firm. Serve.

Nutrition:

calories 243, fat 20.2, fiber 1, carbs 2.8, protein 13.3

Keto Egg Fast Snickerdoodle Crepes

Servings: 2

Cooking Time: 15 Minutes

Ingredients:

- 5 oz cream cheese, softened
- 6 eggs
- 1 teaspoon cinnamon
- Butter, for frying
- 1 tablespoon Swerve
- 2 tablespoons granulated Swerve
- 8 tablespoons butter, softened
- 1 tablespoon cinnamon

Directions:

1. For the crepes: Put all the ingredients together in a blender except the butter and process until smooth.
2. Heat butter on medium heat in a non-stick pan and pour some batter in the pan.
3. Cook for about 2 minutes, then flip and cook for 2 more minutes.
4. Repeat with the remaining mixture.
5. Mix Swerve, butter and cinnamon in a small bowl until combined.
6. Spread this mixture onto the centre of the crepe and serve rolled up.

Nutrition:

Calories: 543 Carbs: 8g Fats: 51.6g Proteins: 15.7g Sodium: 455mg Sugar: 0.9g

Seeds And Lentils Oats

Servings: 4

Cooking Time: 50 Minutes

Ingredients:

- ½ cup red lentils
- ¼ cup pumpkin seeds, toasted
- 2 teaspoons olive oil
- ¼ cup rolled oats
- ¼ cup coconut flesh, shredded
- 1 tablespoon honey
- 1 tablespoon orange zest, grated
- 1 cup Greek yogurt
- 1 cup blackberries

Directions:

1. Spread the lentils on a baking sheet lined with parchment paper, introduce in the oven and roast at 370 degrees F for 30 minutes.
2. Add the rest of the ingredients except the yogurt and the berries, toss and bake at 370 degrees F for 20 minutes more.
3. Transfer this to a bowl, add the rest of the ingredients, toss, divide into smaller bowls and serve for breakfast.

Nutrition:

calories 204, fat 7.1, fiber 10.4, carbs 27.6, protein 9.5

Mediterranean Egg Casserole

Servings:4

Cooking Time:50 Minutes

Ingredients:

Healthy Liver For Life Cookbook

- 1 1/2 cups (6 ounces) feta cheese, crumbled
- 1 jar (6 ounces) marinated artichoke hearts, drained well, coarsely chopped
- 10 eggs
- 2 cups milk, low-fat
- 2 cups fresh baby spinach, packed, coarsely chopped
- 6 cups whole-wheat baguette, cut into 1-inch cubes
- 1 tablespoon garlic (about 4 cloves), finely chopped
- 1 tablespoon olive oil, extra-virgin
- 1/2 cup red bell pepper, chopped
- 1/2 cup Parmesan cheese, shredded

- 1/2 teaspoon pepper
- 1/2 teaspoon red pepper flakes
- 1/2 teaspoon salt
- 1/3 cup kalamata olives, pitted, halved
- 1/4 cup red onion, chopped
- 1/4 cup tomatoes (sun-dried) in oil, drained, chopped

Directions:

1. Preheat oven to 350F.
2. Grease a 9x13-inch baking dish with olive oil cooking spray.
3. In an 8-inch non-stick pan over medium heat, heat the olive oil. Add the onions, garlic, and bell pepper; cook for about 3 minutes, frequently stirring, until slightly softened. Add the spinach; cook for about 1 minute or until starting to wilt.

4. Layer half of the baguette cubes in the preparation ared baking dish, then 1 cup of the eta, 1/4 cup Parmesan, the bell pepper mix, artichokes, the olives, and the tomatoes. Top with the remaining baguette cubes and then with the remaining 1/2 cup of feta.
5. In a large mixing bowl, whisk the eggs and the low-fat milk together. Beat in the pepper, salt and the pepper. Pour the mix over the bread layer in the baking dish, slightly pressing down. Sprinkle with the remaining 1/4 cup Parmesan.
6. Bake for about 40-45 minutes, or until the center is set and the top is golden brown. Before serving, let stand for 15 minutes

Nutrition:

360 Cal, 21 g total fat (9 g sat. fat), 270 mg chol., 880 mg sodium, 24 g carb.,3 g fiber,7 g sugar, 20 g protein.

Red Pepper And Artichoke Frittata

Servings:2

Cooking Time:15 Minutes

Ingredients:

- 4 large eggs
- 1 can (14-ounce) artichoke hearts, rinsed, coarsely chopped
- 1 medium red bell pepper, diced
- 1 teaspoon dried oregano
- 1/4 cup Parmesan cheese, freshly grated
- 1/4 teaspoon red pepper, crushed
- 1/4 teaspoon salt, or to taste
- 2 garlic cloves, minced
- 2 teaspoons extra-virgin olive oil, divided
- Freshly ground pepper, to taste

Directions:

1. In a 10-inch non-stick skillet, heat 1 teaspoon of the olive oil over medium heat. Add the bell pepper; cook for about 2 minutes or until tender. Add the garlic and the red pepper; cook for about 30 seconds, stirring. Transfer the mixture to a plate and wipe the skillet clean.
2. In a medium mixing bowl, whisk the eggs. Stir in the artichokes, cheese, the bell pepper mixture, and season with salt and pepper.
3. Place an over rack 4 inches from the source of heat; preheat broiler.
4. Brush the skillet with the remaining 1 teaspoon olive oil and heat over medium heat. Pour the egg mixture into the skillet and tilt to evenly distribute. Reduce the heat to medium low; cook for about 3-4 minutes, lifting the edges to allow the uncooked egg to flow underneath, until the bottom of the frittata is light golden.
5. Transfer the pan into the broiler, cook for about 1 1/2-2 1/2 minutes, or until the top is set.
6. Slide into a platter; cut into wedges and serve

Nutrition:

305 Cal, 18 g total fat (6 g sat. fat, 8 g mono), 432 mg chol., 734 mg sodium, 1639 mg pot., 18 g carb.,8 g fiber, 21 g protein.

Cinnamon Roll Oats

Servings:4

Cooking Time:10 Minutes

Ingredients:

- ½ cup rolled oats
- 1 cup milk
- 1 teaspoon vanilla extract
- 1 teaspoon ground cinnamon
- 2 teaspoon honey
- 2 tablespoons Plain yogurt
- 1 teaspoon butter

Directions:

1. Pour milk in the saucepan and bring it to boil.
2. Add rolled oats and stir well.
3. Close the lid and simmer the oats for 5 minutes over the medium heat. The cooked oats will absorb all milk.
4. Then add butter and stir the oats well.
5. In the separated bowl, whisk together Plain yogurt with honey, cinnamon, and vanilla extract.
6. Transfer the cooked oats in the serving bowls.
7. Top the oats with the yogurt mixture in the shape of the wheel.

Nutrition:

Calories 243, fat 20.2, fiber 1, carbs 2.8, protein 13.3

Cauliflower Couscous Salad

Servings:4

Cooking Time:25 Minutes

Ingredients:

- 1 large head cauliflower, cut into florets
- 3-4 green onions, thinly sliced
- 2 garlic cloves, finely minced
- 1 jalapeño, seeds and ribs removed, minced
- 1 cup shredded carrots
- 1 cup diced celery
- 1 cup diced cucumber
- 1 green apple, diced
- Juice of 1 lemon
- 1 tablespoon extra-virgin olive oil
- Sea salt
- Freshly ground black peppe

Directions:

1. Using two batches, set your cauliflower to pulse in a food processor until finely chopped.
2. Transfer to a mixing bowl with the remaining ingredients then gently toss until combined.
3. Serve and enjoy.

Nutrition:

3g carbs 10g fat 12g protein 165 Calories

Mediterranean Egg-feta Scramble

Servings: 4

Cooking Time: 20 Minutes

Ingredients:

- 3/4 cup crumbled feta cheese
- 2 tablespoons green onions, minced
- 2 tablespoons red peppers, roasted, diced
- 1/4 teaspoon kosher salt
- 1/4 teaspoon garlic powder
- 1/4 cup Greek yogurt
- 1/2 teaspoon dry oregano
- 1/2 teaspoon dry basil
- 1 teaspoon olive oil
- A few cracks freshly ground black pepper
- Warm whole-wheat tortillas, optional

Directions:

1. Preheat a skillet over medium heat.
2. In a bowl, whisk the eggs, the sour cream, basil, oregano, garlic powder, salt, and pepper. Gently add the feta.
3. When the skillet is hot, add the olive oil and then the egg mixture; allow the egg mix to set then scrape the bottom of the pan to let the uncooked egg to cook. Stir in the red peppers and the green onions. Continue cooking until the eggs mixture is cooked to your preferred doneness. Serve immediately.
4. If desired, sprinkle with extra feta and then wrap the scrambled eggs in tortillas

Nutrition:

260 Cal, 16 g total fat (8 g sat. fat), 350 mg chol., 750 mg sodium, 190 mg pot., 12 g carb.,>1 g fiber, 2 g sugar, 16 g protein.

Detox Porridge

Servings: 2

Cooking Time: 2 Minutes

Ingredients:

- 1 cup unsweetened almond milk
- 2 tablespoons ground golden flax
- 1/2 cup coconut flour
- 1 tablespoon coconut oil
- 1 teaspoon cinnamon
- 1 cup water
- 1 tablespoon raw honey
- Toasted coconut to serve
- Toasted almonds to serve

Directions:

1. In a microwave safe bowl, stir together all the ingredients until well combined; place in the microwave and heat for 1 minute.
2. Stir again to mix well and microwave for another 1 minute. Serve right away topped with toasted almonds and toasted coconut.

Nutrition:

242 Calories 7g Carbs 19g Fat 12g Protein

Mexican Style Burritos

Servings:2

Cooking Time:15 Minutes

Ingredients:

- Olive oil – 1 Tablespoon
- Corn tortillas – 2
- Red onion – ¼ cup, chopped
- Red bell peppers – ¼ cup, chopped
- Red chili – ½, deseeded and chopped
- Eggs – 2
- Juice of 1 lime
- Cilantro – 1 Tablespoon chopped

Directions:

1. Turn the broiler to medium heat and place the tortillas underneath for 1 to 2 minutes on each side or until lightly toasted.
2. Remove and keep the broiler on.
3. Sauté onion, chili and bell peppers for 5 to 6 minutes or until soft.
4. Place the eggs on top of the onions and peppers and place skillet under the broiler for 5-6 minutes or until the eggs are cooked.
5. Serve half the eggs and vegetables on top of each tortilla and sprinkle with cilantro and lime juice to serve

Nutrition:

Calories: 202 ,Fat: 13g ,Carb: 19g ,Phosphorus: 184mg ,Potassium: 233mg ,Sodium: 77mg ,Protein: 9g

Stuffed Figs

Servings: 2

Cooking Time: 15 Minutes

Ingredients:

- 7 oz fresh figs
- 1 tablespoon cream cheese
- ½ teaspoon walnuts, chopped
- 4 bacon slices
- ¼ teaspoon paprika
- ¼ teaspoon salt
- ½ teaspoon canola oil
- ½ teaspoon honey

Directions:

1. Make the crosswise cuts in every fig.
2. In the shallow bowl mix up together cream cheese, walnuts, paprika, and salt.
3. Fill the figs with cream cheese mixture and wrap in the bacon.
4. Secure the fruits with toothpicks and sprinkle with honey.
5. Line the baking tray with baking paper.
6. Place the preparation ared figs in the tray and sprinkle them with olive oil gently.
7. Bake the figs for 15 minutes at 350F.

Nutrition:

Calories 299, fat 19.4, fiber 2.3, carbs 16.7, protein 15.2

Tapioca Pudding

Servings: 3

Cooking Time: 15 Minutes

Ingredients:

- ¼ cup pearl tapioca
- ¼ cup maple syrup
- 2 cups almond milk
- ½ cup coconut flesh, shredded
- 1 and ½ teaspoon lemon juice

Directions:

1. In a pan, combine the milk with the tapioca and the rest of the ingredients, bring to a simmer over medium heat, and cook for 15 minutes.
2. Divide the mix into bowls, cool it down and serve for breakfast.

Nutrition:

calories 361, fat 28.5, fiber 2.7, carbs 28.3, protein 2.8

Pumpkin Muffins

Servings:12

Cooking Time:20 Minutes

Ingredients:

- 1 cup all-purpose flour
- 1 cup wheat bran
- 2 teaspoons Phosphorus Powder
- 1 cup pumpkin purée
- ¼ cup honey
- ¼ cup olive oil
- 1 egg
- 1 teaspoon vanilla extract
- ½ cup cored diced apple

Directions:

1. Preheat the oven to 400°F.
2. Line 12 muffin cups with paper liners.
3. Stir together the flour, wheat bran, and baking powder, mix this in a medium bowl.
4. In a small bowl, whisk together the pumpkin, honey, olive oil, egg, and vanilla.
5. Stir the pumpkin mixture into the flour mixture until just combined.
6. Stir in the diced apple.
7. Spoon the batter in the muffin cups.
8. Bake for about 20 minutes, or until a toothpick inserted in the center of a muffin comes out clean.

Nutrition:

Calories: 125; Total Fat: 5g; Saturated Fat: 1g; Cholesterol: 18mg; Sodium: 8mg; Carbohydrates: 20g; Fiber: 3g; Phosphorus: 120mg; Potassium: 177mg; Protein: 2g

Snack

Za'atar Fries

Servings:3

Cooking Time:35 Minutes

Ingredients:

- 1 teaspoon Za'atar spices
- 3 sweet potatoes
- 1 tablespoon dried dill
- 1 teaspoon salt
- 3 teaspoons sunflower oil
- ½ teaspoon paprika

Directions:

1. Pour water in the crockpot. Peel the sweet potatoes and cut them into the fries.
2. Line the baking tray with parchment.
3. Place the layer of the sweet potato in the tray.
4. Sprinkle the vegetables with dried dill, salt, and paprika.
5. Then sprinkle sweet potatoes with Za'atar and mix up well with the help of the fingertips.
6. Sprinkle the sweet potato fries with sunflower oil.
7. Preheat the oven to 375F.
8. Bake the sweet potato fries for 35 minutes. Stir the fries every 10 minutes.

Nutrition:

calories 28, fat 2.9, fiber 0.2, carbs 0.6, protein 0.2

Orange Salsa

Servings:3

Cooking Time:30 Minutes

Ingredients:

- 1½ C. fresh mango, cut into chunks
- 1½ C. fresh pineapple, peeled, pitted and cubed
- ¼ C. red onion, chopped
- 2 tbsp. fresh cilantro, chopped
- 2 tbsp. fresh orange juice
- Salt and freshly ground black pepper, to taste
- 2 tbsp. unsweetened coconut, shredded

Directions:

1. In a large bowl, add all ingredients except coconut and gently toss to coat well.
2. Serve immediately with the topping of coconut.

Nutrition:

448 Calories 27g fat 41g carbs 15g protein

Crazy Saganaki Shrimp

Servings: 4

Cooking Time: 10 Minutes

Ingredients:

- ¼ tsp salt
- ½ cup Chardonnay
- ½ cup crumbled Greek feta cheese
- 1 medium bulb. fennel, cored and finely chopped
- 1 small Chile pepper, seeded and minced
- 1 tbsp extra virgin olive oil
- 12 jumbo shrimps, peeled and deveined with tails left on
- 2 tbsp lemon juice, divided
- 5 scallions sliced thinly
- Pepper to taste

Directions:

1. In medium bowl, mix salt, lemon juice and shrimp.
2. On medium fire, place a saganaki pan (or large nonstick saucepan) and heat oil.
3. Sauté Chile pepper, scallions, and fennel for 4 minutes or until starting to brown and is already soft.
4. Add wine and sauté for another minute.
5. Place shrimps on top of fennel, cover and cook for 4 minutes or until shrimps are pink.
6. Remove just the shrimp and transfer to a plate.
7. Add pepper, feta and 1 tbsp lemon juice to pan and cook for a minute or until cheese begins to melt.
8. To serve, place cheese and fennel mixture on a serving plate and top with shrimps.

Nutrition:

Calories per serving: 310; Protein: 49.7g; Fat: 6.8g; Carbs: 8.4g

Apple Chips

Servings: 4

Cooking Time: 45 Minutes

Ingredients:

- 2 Golden Delicious apples, cored and thinly sliced
- 1 1/2 teaspoons white sugar
- 1/2 teaspoon ground cinnamon

Directions:

1. Set your oven to 225 degrees F.
2. Place apple slices on a baking sheet.
3. Sprinkle sugar an
4. d cinnamon over apple slices.
5. Bake for 45 minutes.
6. Serve

Nutrition:

Calories 127 ,Total Fat 3.5 g ,Saturated Fat 0.5 g ,Cholesterol 162 mg ,Sodium 142 mg ,Total Carbs 33.6g ,Fiber 0.4 g ,Sugar 0.5 g ,Protein 4.5 g

Walnut & Spiced Apple Tonic

Servings: 1

Cooking Time: 15 Minutes

Ingredients:

- 6 walnuts halves
- 1 apple, cored
- 1 banana
- ½ teaspoon matcha powder
- ½ teaspoon cinnamon
- Pinch of ground nutmeg

Directions:

1. Place ingredients into a blender and add sufficient water to cover them. Blitz until smooth and creamy.

Nutrition:

Calories: 124 ,Sodium: 22 mg ,Dietary Fiber: 1.4 g ,Total Fat: 2.1 g ,Total Carbs: 12.3 g ,Protein: 1.2 g

Raw Broccoli Poppers

Servings: 4

Cooking Time: 8 Minutes

Ingredients:

- 1/8 cup water
- 1/8 tsp. fine sea salt
- 4 cups broccoli florets, washed and cut into 1-inch pieces
- 1/4 tsp. turmeric powder
- 1 cup unsalted cashews, soaked overnight or at least 3-4 hours and drained
- 1/4 tsp. onion powder
- 1 red bell pepper, seeded and
- 2 tbsp. nutritional heaping
- 2 tbsp. lemon juice

Directions:

1. Transfer the drained cashews to a high-speed blender and pulse for about 30 seconds. Add in the chopped pepper and pulse again for 30 seconds.
2. Add 2 tbsp. of lemon juice, 1/8 cup of water, 2 tbsp. of nutritional yeast/ heaping, ¼ tsp. of onion powder, 1/8 of tsp. fine sea salt, and 1/4 tsp. of turmeric powder. Pulse for about 45 seconds until smooth.
3. Handover the broccoli into a bowl and add in the chopped cheesy cashew mixture. Toss well until coated.
4. Transfer the pieces of broccoli to the trays of a yeast dehydrator.
5. Follow the dehydrator's instructions and dehydrate for about 8 minutes at 125°F or until crunchy.

Nutrition:

Calories: 408 .Fats: 32 g ,Carbs: 22 g ,Protein: 15 g

Cod And Cabbage

Servings:4

Cooking Time:15 Minutes

Ingredients:

- 3 cups green cabbage, shredded
- 1 sweet onion, sliced
- A pinch of salt and black pepper
- ½ cup feta cheese, crumbled
- 4 teaspoons olive oil
- 4 cod fillets, boneless
- ¼ cup green olives, pitted and chopped

Directions:

1. Grease a roasting pan with the oil, add the fish, the cabbage and the rest of the ingredients, introduce in the pan and cook at 450 degrees F for 15 minutes.
2. Divide the mix between plates and serve

Nutrition:

calories 270, fat 10, fiber 3, carbs 12, protein 31

Healthy Carrot & Shrimp

Servings: 4

Cooking Time: 30 Minutes

Ingredients:

- 1 lb shrimp, peeled and deveined
- 1 tbsp chives, chopped
- 1 onion, chopped
- 1 tbsp olive oil
- 1 cup fish stock
- 1 cup carrots, sliced
- Pepper
- Salt

Directions:

1. Add oil into the inner pot of instant pot and set the pot on sauté mode.
2. Add onion and sauté for 2 minutes.
3. Add shrimp and stir well.
4. Add remaining ingredients and stir well.
5. Seal pot with lid and cook on high for 4 minutes.
6. Once done, release pressure using quick release. Remove lid.
7. Serve and enjoy.

Nutrition:

Calories 197 Fat 5.9 g Carbohydrates 7 g Sugar 2.5 g Protein 27.7 g Cholesterol 239 mg

Spiced Toasted Almonds & Seed Mix

Servings: 4

Cooking Time: 10 Minutes

Ingredients:

- 2 tablespoons olive oil
- 1/2 cup sunflower seeds
- 1/2 cup pumpkin seeds
- 1 cup almonds
- 1 tablespoon chili paste
- 1 tablespoon crushed fennel seeds
- 1 tablespoon ground cumin
- ½ teaspoon sea salt

Directions:

1. Heat oil in a skillet set over medium heat; stir in chili paste and fennel seeds and then add in seeds and almonds; sauté for about 5 minutes and then stir in cumin and salt. Remove from heat and let cool before servin

Nutrition:

448 Calories 27g fat 41g carbs 15g protein

Conclusion

Eating can improve and alleviate symptoms of liver cirrhosis. It is important to stay hydrated with water, juice or other fluids because dehydration will cause a build up of toxins in the body. A diet low in fat but high in protein and carbohydrates help maintain proper weight while giving essential nutrients for fighting off infection. The list goes on! But one thing that you need to know about your liver is that it's still working hard even if you have lost 80% function due to alcohol abuse.

Healthy Liver For Life Cookbook

Cirrhosis is an irreversible, chronic liver disease that can lead to complete organ failure. The cirrhosis diet plays a major role in the course of this condition and there are both eating tips for people with liver cirrhosis as well as information on how the functions of the liver work. You're not alone; many people suffer from this disease without knowing they are living with it until later stages when the risks increase considerably, so let's take care of our livers so we can live better!

www.ingramcontent.com/pod-product-compliance
Lightning Source LLC
Chambersburg PA
CBHW070914080526
44589CB00013B/1292